Embracing a New Vision of Aging

EMBRACING
A NEW VISION OF
AGING

SHERYL TOWERS

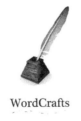

WordCrafts

Published by WordCrafts Press
Cody, Wyoming 82414
www.wordcrafts.net

For my son, Justin.

Contents

Questioning Societal Attitudes

A positive and life-affirming perception of aging is taking root in our culture, and a much-needed shift is emerging. A cultural shift that is embracing aging with creativity and gratitude, and moving towards exploring the possibilities of our increased life span, is slowly gathering momentum. We are breaking through to new levels of awareness and personal power as we challenge old fears and outdated ways of perceiving aging. In many ways, we are claiming the power to make up our own rules and to say good-bye to the conventional stereotypes and limitations.

Though this social tipping point reflects how far our views of aging have come, they have not come far enough. We need to make further advances in embracing this unprecedented opportunity to socially construct the aging process so that it is an enriching model for all.

In spite of our progress, our culture continues to transmit the negative message that aging is to be dreaded and denied. Our minds continue to be crammed by the media with the dreadful data of age-related scenarios proclaiming that aging is a collection of diseases and losses. These cultural perspectives foster a fear of aging in our society which has become a pronounced syndrome that dramatically affects our experience of growing older.

The fear of aging isn't a recent phenomenon as the idea of the fountain of youth and methods of rejuvenation can be traced through the centuries. What is different today, though, is how these anxieties are reinforced by mass media and how early anxieties about aging begin. Given that we are living longer and that the potential length of our life span is still in question, unless we experience an even greater shift in our consciousness, this means that we are going to be worried for a long time.

In the last hundred years, the average life expectancy has dramatically increased, but for many the later years have not been a time of happiness and well-being. Having been culturally indoctrinated to fear a long decline, many dread their potential for a longer life rather than embracing this new longevity. This paradigm of aging is false and limiting. The time has come to challenge the myth of decline and to celebrate our new gift of longevity which is truly wondrous. The time has come to explore the steady emergence of the new possibilities and capacities which aging offers and to discover what use we are to make of our extended life span.

The truth is that we weren't created to blossom early and then spend the rest of our life withering away. The more we learn about aging, the more we know that a sweeping downward trajectory is grossly inadequate. The path of our aging is not written in stone or even in our ancestry. We have the potential to grow older free of disease and disability and to function well both cognitively and physically.

The reality is that there is tremendous variability in how we age that primarily stems from lifestyle choices and attitude. Even if certain health conditions run in our family, there is much we can do to break those patterns. For most of us, a healthy lifestyle trumps inherited risk. In fact, the majority of the ingredients that predict longevity and good health are within our control.

For example, recent research shows that some areas of the brain involved with memory and learning continue to produce new nerve cells every day. So while we do lose brain cells on a daily basis, we also are constantly replacing them. We can build new brain cells by keeping our brain active with new activities and learning.

Research also shows that most disease-related gene mutations are influenced by lifestyle including emotions, stress levels, diet, and quality of sleep. In addition, the new science of epigenetics tells us that we may have much more control over the cellular biology of our aging than we otherwise thought. Questions remain at the most basic level about what triggers aging in our bodies, why it occurs and what the biological processes are that underlie these changes.

We are also learning that we have a chronological age and a biological age. While our chronological age reflects the age on our birth certificate, our biological age basically reflects how well our body is functioning. Our biological age doesn't always match our chronological age and is determined by, among other things, our expectations and beliefs, our perception of the aging process, and our energy level. We can be much younger or older than the age stated on our birth certificate.

However, despite reams of research countering the false narratives spun by the myths of aging, they persist. Society's long-held projection of aging as an inexorable process of decline makes bypassing this fear a bold challenge. We do have the power, however, to take on this challenge. We can leave behind these damaging stereotypes which restrict our happiness and freedom, and choose those beliefs that are in alignment with our highest potential.

We can accept the process of growing older which is the inevitable process of moving through life along the time continuum without experiencing it as a signal of decline in our health or enjoyment of life. Growing older is a physical process, whereas getting old is a mental and spiritual one heavily influenced by our culture and its stereotypes.

Spirit and attitude play a large part in the concept of being old. Being old is hanging onto old ideas and beliefs that no longer work and living in the past. Being old is focusing on what you can't do rather than what you can do, and getting lost in playing the part of the victim. Being old is focusing on the losses rather than the possibilities.

Aging, just like the rest of life, is a mixture of gains and losses, but the gains associated with aging are hidden in our culture. As a culture, we have generally approached aging from a negative attitude viewing it as the loss of all the good things youth offers and seeing it only as the diminishing of our physical body. Though our physical body will age and our physical appearance will change, our minds and spirits do not have to age.

Changing our attitude can help move us from the declinist vision of aging which has permeated our culture to viewing aging as growth—as a daring path toward our authentic self. This attitude shift can help us see our later years as an opportunity to fully mature and actualize our creative potential, to see these years as, in fact, the most powerful and satisfying phase of our life. We can use these years to realize the purpose for which we were born.

We can have a wonderful life in youth, and we can have a wonderful life in our later years. The choice is ours as we are the pioneers redefining aging. We must blaze our own trail rather than have it created for us by others. Whatever our future will be is largely a personal choice based on the stories we tell ourselves. Regardless of the media influences or cultural pressures that can make us feel negative about growing older, our own self-perceptions about aging are in the locus of our control.

Research has identified that our self-perceptions about getting older can create a self-fulfilling prophecy. Negative perceptions about aging can have a detrimental effect on both our physical and cognitive health. Positive perceptions help us see the value that aging offers—particularly to the creative and spiritual dimensions of our life.

Recognizing that shifting words can shift perceptions, researchers are presenting many new aging concepts such as successful aging, conscious aging, positive aging and even anti-aging. These new labels have the intention of inspiring us to see growing older differently than we do now, allowing us to create a new story around our aging process.

Breaking the traditional notions of aging, as well as refusing to buy into the prejudicial attitudes, is up to each one of us. When we can see the prison in which we have put ourselves, we can also see our potential. Ageism is a prison, and it is alive and operating at every level of our society. We must be careful not to buy into this cultural model. As each of us embraces a new vision of aging for ourselves, we have the opportunity to create a new cultural paradigm which will serve generations to come.

2

Modeling Positive Messages
For Our Children

Children's chances of surviving to a very old age are greater than at any time in history. Given this longevity, they need a perspective which promotes positive expectations of aging as a natural, desirable, lifelong process of growth and development to be honored. They need an understanding of old age that offers the opportunity for meaning and fulfillment throughout the course of their lives.

Unfortunately, influenced by the media and what they see and hear in everyday life, children tend to develop negative stereotypes about aging. Far too often they see older adults portrayed as dependent, unproductive, helpless and demanding. These stereotypes typically persist as children grow up leaving them completely unaware that they have acquired or accepted these attitudes. With this lack of awareness, they grow into old age assuming the stereotypes to be true and living them out. Thus the negative stereotypes acquired in childhood parade across the adult life span as expectations.

We don't want our children to develop negative expectations

about what will happen to them as a result of being old, or how it will feel to be old. Turning around the widely held negative attitudes, beliefs, and stereotypes based on chronological age is up to each one of us. Otherwise, taking the ingrained ageism in stride and unconsciously passing it on to our children allows the limitations and suffering of these biases to persist.

As we develop a greater understanding as to how our attitude toward aging will either be a blessing or a curse upon the coming generations, we can choose to deconstruct those beliefs and myths that are restrictive and disempowering and do not help mold the lives of our children in a positive way. Dispelling the myths can help change the stereotypical views and liberate us to see new possibilities.

The most important way to dispel the myths is for each of us to be a positive role model. The way we move through aging molds the emotional attitudes of the younger people within the orbit of our influence. Children spend a great deal of time observing the attitudes of those around them and usually begin to demonstrate similar outlooks as well as to imitate those close to them. If they hear their parents talking negatively or chronically complaining about aging, this can generate feelings of dread and fear as well as prevent them from enjoying the natural and rewarding process of aging.

Children must be able to see older people in a favorable way in order to develop positive feelings toward their own age and the aging process. They must see how creatively, adventurously, and optimistically adults live life so they will be happy about growing up themselves. They need to see older adults living lives that are beyond the popular stereotype of loneliness, senility and eccentric behavior.

Seeing positive models of older adults and positive images of aging lays a foundation for successful living for children in their later years. To the contrary, portrayals of the misery and illness of older people set up the expectation that aging is something to be feared and perpetuates a negative image of the later years.

Since perceptions of aging begin to form early in life, it is essential that education about aging starts at a young age. Such education would minimize the possibility of ageist attitudes developing as well as the likelihood of internalizing fear about the aging process. It would also provide children with guidance as to how to live out their entire life span as healthy, productive, effective individuals. Ideally this education would translate into healthier habits and lifestyle choices that increase the chances of maintaining good health and vigor throughout their life. Education would teach young people that while aging is inevitable, how we age is largely up to us.

Before we can effectively teach children, we must confront our own fears and stereotypes about aging. We must see how our own perceptions of aging influence our interactions with older people. Age is so stigmatized in our culture that we tend to dis-identify with older people. In fact, many of us do not even want to be around older people which often leads to marginalizing, ignoring, and even reviling the elderly. We don't want to face what we are so afraid we will become. We are uncomfortable being around people who are walking examples of the fact that we will all eventually get old and die.

Distancing and dis-identifying with older people is aided by the shift in family lifestyles. The family lifestyle of today has resulted in more segregation and less frequent interaction between children and older adults. In many ways we have become an age-segregated society in which we cluster into age groups, particularly in our later years. In the absence of this exceedingly important intergenerational connecting, myths and stereotypes have the potential to flourish. A promising route to the reduction of negative stereotypes and attitudes is more frequent and positive intergenerational connecting.

Another promising route to the reduction of negative stereotypes is already being seen as a result primarily of the longevity explosion, medical research, and baby boomer expectations. Positive societal messages are emerging making vitality and personal growth the new normal of aging. The way advertisers are beginning to promote to the more mature generation reflects this new normal. Companies are now re-shaping their products and marketing strategies as they are becoming aware that older people are very active, want to explore, learn new things, and venture out into new endeavors. Marketers are showing more creativity and respect for the ever-evolving senior generation who are consistently learning and creating new values for themselves. Businesses are learning to appreciate rather than depreciate this growing population.

As we yearn for a society in which we can all grow older graciously, fearlessly, and together, we need to create even more positive messages. We need to model for our children that every year of a long life allows us the opportunity to cultivate a lively, curious, creative, and cultured mind. We need to teach our children not to focus on the mere physical manifestations of aging but on what cannot be taken away: the love we give and receive and the wisdom we have gained.

We need to help the younger generations understand the deeper meanings of life which come from attaining our own wholeness and wisdom first. We do this by choosing to live each moment growing more aware and wiser. We do this by approaching our life-to its very end-filled with awe and striving to offer something of value for those coming after us. We do this with an awareness that our words and deeds will affect those whom we will never see.

3

Healing Age Shame

We often notice that the first piece of information in a news article, right after a person's name, is their age. This is a clue as to how society defines age as such a crucial feature of a person's identity. Clearly, age is one of the countless methods used to size people up, to determine the expectations of them, and to put them in a specific box. In other words, while perhaps not consciously realizing we are doing so, we utilize age as one of the factors by which we judge each other and ourselves.

The truth is that age has very little to do with who we truly are or what we stand for in life despite the fact that our culture insists on assigning significant value to it. In fact, age is not a good indication of very much about us except identifying the number of years we have been given to experience this journey on earth. The calendar simply tells us what our chronological age is, a number that is far from accurate in defining anything noteworthy about us.

The time has come to give up the grip which this number has over our self-image and sense of possibilities, and to cast aside this narrow and imprecise measure of our identity. The

time has come to do our own thinking, unfettered by the attitudes of others, and allow a whole new range of possibilities
and freedom to open up to us regardless of our age. As we
challenge both those external and internal forces that we allow
to limit our potential as we age, we begin to liberate ourselves
from the mass hypnosis that this deep- seated cultural conditioning has created.

Breaking through the stereotypes means first of all becoming
aware of any thoughts and behaviors which reveal our core
beliefs around aging. We need to see what is hidden inside us
so that we don't blindly repeat these limiting judgments. We
can begin by noticing if we tend to collude with the disempowering idea that older is lesser which convinces us that we
are less valuable with each passing birthday. We can notice if
we tend to judge ourselves by the cultural standard of equating
worth with youth and youthful beauty.

We can observe if we are treating our age like a shameful
secret because we want to avoid the stigma that growing older
in today's world brings. We can become aware that withhold-
ing or lying about our age (or even whispering our age in
secret), reveals a subtle but shame-based attitude towards aging
that may not even be in our conscious awareness. We can also
become aware that choosing to engage in these behaviors feeds
the notion that there is something dreadful about aging –something inferior or shameful about growing older.

As we work to become more aware of our own attitudes
toward aging, we also need to have compassion for ourselves for
not wanting to be seen as old in our youth-worshiping culture.
Being seen as old carries a lot of baggage in our society; thus, it
is no wonder that we feel vulnerable and uncomfortable telling
our age. In fact, women have been taught to conceal their age
and even lie about it. This secretiveness is not only disempowering, but it also generates an unnecessary and subtle guilt

about no longer being young. The emotion of guilt is generated when we judge ourselves as being in the "wrong." Society's aversion to aging can generate these feelings of being in the wrong because older people are seen as far removed from the cultural ideals. Feeling far removed from the ideal can make it difficult for us to keep our head held high and can set us up to get caught in the shame cycle.

Shame about aging is in great part a result of the ageism which exists in our society. In many ways this prejudice is considered socially accepted as demonstrated by the ideas presented in jokes, birthday cards, and the media representing older people as frail, incompetent, cranky, senile, inferior and even laughable. These images and notions permeate our culture so thoroughly that their biased messages often slip by us.

Ageist sentiments are very subtle in nature and can even appear on the surface as a compliment—although they are patronizing and often condescending. For example, addressing an older woman as young lady perpetuates the idea that old is bad and young is good. To be addressed in such a way would only be flattering and make us feel pleased if we did believe that young is better than old.

These stereotypes generate negative self-perceptions which feed our fears and erode our confidence. In fact, at its core shame is an attachment to a negative self-perception that has been fostered by the opinions of others. This shame causes us to feel fearful and vulnerable, and it generates feelings of being unworthy, inferior, and unlovable-all of which distort our sense of self. Sadly, these feelings describe what it is like for so many of us to reveal and deal with our age, particularly when our self-worth is bound up with the worth we perceive we have in the eyes of others.

There is real danger in allowing the reactions of others to our age to determine how we feel about ourselves and our sense of worth. If we allow a label that others stamp on us because of our age and their own prejudices to become our reality, we put our personal power right into their hands. Only when the perceptions held by others becomes less important to us will we be able to be our true self and appreciate our worth. As we do so, an immense amount of stress and worry falls away while an immense sense of freedom surfaces.

The truth is we can't expect people to respect our age when we don't respect it ourselves. Until we transcend our disempowering beliefs and stop behaving in self-sabotaging ways, the signs of denial and anxiety over aging will permeate every aspect of our lives albeit very subtly. To be free, we must make a decision to cease believing things about ourselves that make us feel bad and to stop behaving in ways that perpetuate our fears. Otherwise, we will experience a loss of self-confidence, a lack of motivation, and a pessimism about the future which will all profoundly influence our health and longevity as well as our self-concept and what we see as our possibilities.

Pessimistic perspectives of aging cause us to engage in negative self-talk and say things to ourselves we would never dream of saying to someone we care about. For instance, it is doubtful we would call a friend old and ugly, or tell them they didn't measure up, or say anything that would cause them to devalue themselves. Yet, buying into the negative views and images with which we have been programmed causes us to judge and reject ourselves. Making a conscious choice to break free of this negative programming allows us to claim the power to make up our own rules and to embrace our potential. Otherwise, envisioning a life of great possibilities is not within our capacity when our mind is filled with these pessimistic thoughts.

Our responsibility is to challenge these unhelpful aspects of our thinking by questioning their validity and replacing them with more reasonable and constructive thoughts. Our opportunity is to define what aging means to us and to refuse to use age as an excuse to hold ourselves back. As we embrace and appreciate our age, we experience a shift in our consciousness which reflects a new mindset in how we see the process of aging and ourselves. We then let go of our old ways of reacting which includes any hesitation about sharing our age.

By choosing to let go of our hesitancy to openly share our age, we step out of shame and take a stand in living a life that is a reflection of our own authentic self. This might require that we be vulnerable and dare to break away from the security of our comfort zone, but until we do so, the shame associated with aging will persist.

It often takes just a single brave person to change the trajectory of a cultural pattern. In fact, changing stereotypes is largely the job of each of us individually. When even one of us refuses to buy into the societal messages that prey on our fears and separates us from our sense of worthiness and personal power, we help all to become liberated. At the same time, when we buy into the negative beliefs, we make it more difficult for others to break through.

Sadly, one of the most subtle and deeply held negative beliefs is that we lose our worth as we get older. This erosion of self-worth is particularly pronounced in later life as we experience increasing changes in our roles, relationships and physical health. However, it is entirely possible to navigate through these changes with our self-worth intact, for certainly we do not lose our worth as we get older – we can't lose our worth. But if we believe we do, we feel full of fear and insecurities as our emotional reactions are congruent with our deeply held beliefs.

The good news is that our beliefs can be altered and we can choose ones that serve us better. We can find a refreshing sense of freedom by looking at the programs which have been driving our life and by being willing to let go of any outdated or erroneous scripts we've been handed. Healing and transforming whatever negativity and fear we harbor within about aging is a wonderful gift to ourselves. We cannot experience the joy of being who we truly are until we are comfortable with our age. Pretending, hiding and feeling shameful are such detriments to our spirit while courage and honesty transform us.

As we accept the truth that many of the ideas we have about age are long past their expiration date, we can help bring forth an age-acceptance movement that embraces the gift of growing older. Ideas are contagious and control our destiny. They gradually spread until whole cultures are influenced by them. New ideas produce new behavior, and behavioral changes of the people in society foster cultural change.

The time is ripe to cultivate new ideas about the possibilities of aging and to leave behind our phobia and shame. The time has come to look at all those aspects of aging which frighten us and to give aging a new, life-affirming meaning.

4

Understanding the Power of Belief

Aging in itself does not close us off and limit our world, but our negative beliefs do. We have so many ideas about aging—about what it means and what it looks like—that do not serve us well. Many of these beliefs are assumptions which were constructed on social norms and expectations that are no longer valid. In fact, the majority of the expectations of the aging process were created long ago by people living in a very different environment than what we live in today.

For example, disease, disability, and dependency were once considered an inevitable part of growing older, but today we know this is not necessarily our destiny. Though aging can put us at a greater risk for health issues, we have the potential to live healthy, active and independent lives well into our advanced years as many older people are currently modeling. Another example of an outdated belief about aging, as mentioned in chapter one, is the idea that adults can't improve their brain function. This assumption has been uprooted with recent research revealing the fact that we can continuously grow new brain cells, or neurons, throughout our life.

Yet, even with increasing data debunking ideas which no longer hold true, many of the assumptions about aging are still believed by the masses. The cultural conditioning is so strong that far too many of us continue to be convinced that life must unfold in a certain way, and typically that is a downhill trajectory. Unfortunately, myths about aging have become crystallized into immutable beliefs.

These deeply rooted convictions about the aging process and about ourselves significantly influence our thoughts and actions. In fact, our beliefs about anything actually serve as the building blocks of our life and are the filters through which we interpret our experiences. Furthermore, the experiences of our life are fundamentally and primarily the external representation of the inner beliefs and conversations we have within ourselves. Essentially, what we believe is what we experience.

The self-fulfilling prophecy of our deep-seated convictions can be revealed when we are able to make the connection between our internal beliefs and our external experiences. For example, if we hold the belief that aging narrows our opportunities, we can observe how this plays out in our life. We can notice in what areas of our life we hold ourselves back due to this belief and thus prevent ourselves from being proactive in pursuing those things which would bring us fulfillment.

Another example would be to notice if we primarily believe the world is a place of promise and possibility, which is necessary in order to see our opportunities, or if we view life as predominantly about obstacles, problems, and limitations. We can discern if we have the belief that aging will change us for the worse and believe that we have no power over the process. If so, we can observe how this belief results in feelings of helplessness and hopelessness, and how those feelings affect our emotional well-being.

One of the ways to discover our beliefs is through paying

attention to our conversations, as the words we speak come forth as an automatic reaction of our belief system. What and how we say things to others and to ourselves is a direct result of our thought processes based on our beliefs which create our map of reality. For example, the statement "I am having a senior moment" reveals the expectation that losing our memory is inherent in aging.

When we reply with the familiar cliché "You can't teach an old dog new tricks," we see another example of an underlying belief surfacing. Inherit in this trite phrase is the idea that older people aren't able or willing to change their established patterns of opinion or behavior. These comments reflect unquestioned beliefs which are negative and limiting. The good news is that we can make a conscious choice to see things from a different perspective as we become more aware.

Gaining insight into our beliefs through self-observation allows us to begin to discern and make new choices. We can begin to question what our mind is telling us rather than to totally identify with our thoughts. We can discover just how untrue and untrustworthy our thoughts can be and realize that we don't have to believe everything they tell us. We can discover that much of what we hold to be true is not a conscious choice. Instead, it is derived from long-established and unchallenged habits of thinking.

Developing these skills of observation and questioning are the first steps to changing any beliefs that no longer serve us. In taking these steps, we can become more self-determined and less at the mercy of our old habits and mind conditioning. We can then break free of unexamined patterns of thinking that do not work for us by inquiring as to their validity and by asserting ourselves to be the creator of our own habits of thought. Breaking free of these patterns requires staying committed to living consciously; otherwise we operate automatically.

Unfortunately, attempting to live consciously is indeed counteracted by the heavy unconsciousness of the world in which we live. Whether we are aware of it or not, we are all victims of cultural conditioning, in many instances to the point of being hypnotized. Choosing empowering beliefs about aging can be extremely challenging when each day we are bombarded by magazine articles, media advertisements, and other images depicting the negative experiences of growing older. These negative stereotypes of aging are so deeply ingrained that they can feel almost impossible to overcome. We can, however, refuse to be a victim of this mass thinking or to feed upon the suggestions of others as we choose to live through our own volition and intentions.

If we do not change our negative habits of thinking about aging, each passing birthday will be a threat, and the disempowering stories we tell ourselves will continue to exert their strong influence. And each time we tell ourselves these demoralizing stories, we reinforce them. To break through this self-defeating cycle, we must choose to change the stories that no longer serve our personal or cultural evolution rather than to be bound to their limiting consequences. We must be willing to change our minds in order to change our lives.

In short, we need to stop misusing the power of our mind by refusing to engage in negative and fearful images of aging. Anxiety producing stories about aging which fill us with dread and worry lead to using our imagination to think about and visualize what we fear rather than what we desire. These fearful thoughts are just as creative and magnetic in attracting difficulties to us as are the constructive thoughts in attracting positive outcomes. They can become a self-fulfilling prophecy and be the single most powerful agent in creating exactly what we fear.

Some of the most renowned experiments on the occurrence of a self-fulfilling prophecy are those involving the placebo effect. A placebo is an inert, innocuous substance that has no effect on the body. Yet when patients are given the placebo believing they are getting an actual drug, they subsequently feel better, despite receiving no actual treatment at all. The placebo is considered an expectation effect, and demonstrates how our expectations, emotions, and thoughts contribute to what we experience.

Of course, just as the mind can make things better, it can also make things worse. The nocebo effect is the flip side of the placebo effect in that it generates a negative reaction.

The reason the placebo and nocebo effects are important is that they reveal the power of expectations and are examples of how our mind can shape our reality. In fact, expectations so powerfully affect the experience of our life that we could say our expectations are the coming attractions of our lives.

Our expectations about aging have more to do with what we experience than the actual process of aging. If not, then everyone would respond to the aging process the same, yet we witness dramatic differences. Establishing the intention to adopt age-positive expectations and behaviors enhances our ability to flourish on our aging journey. In addition, creating a cocoon of positive expectancy for ourselves by surrounding ourselves with ideas and people who share our positive intentions strengthens our optimism.

Being optimistic is difficult if we believe our best days are behind us. If we anticipate our later years as some unwanted future experience or obsess about the worst case scenarios of getting older, we only generate pessimism. By doing so we cause our bodies to already be living in that stressful reality. Making the conscious decision to change our beliefs to a new and more promising way of looking at aging not only insures a happier future, but also contributes to our current emotional well-being.

Rather than obsessing about the negative changes of aging

that we fear, a more powerful stance is to focus upon what we desire to experience, embrace it emotionally, and take action to make it happen. Consistently maintaining this focus with positive expectation enables us to create a happy life for ourselves for all the days of our life, and provides a strong foundation for growing older in great health, with vibrant energy, and with our brain intact.

As we whole-heartedly believe that wonderful and adventurous things are possible for us, we will come to expect, not just wish, for the best. We will come to see that growing older does not have to mean a loss of the excitement and pleasure that we experienced in our youth, nor does it mean we must abandon our dreams. We have both the ability and responsibility to ignore those cultural beliefs that prevent us from pursuing our dreams. As we claim our personal power and choose to create our own empowering stories and positive expectations, we develop a stronger will and a greater resiliency to handle the challenges that come our way.

5

CRAFTING EMOTIONAL RESILIENCE

Aging means change. Some of the changes we experience with aging can create feelings of loss of control, as if we have been abducted into an unwelcome phase of life. The changes in our physical body, the death of people close to us, the adaptation to new technology, and other life experiences can cause us to feel vulnerable and defenseless. The good news is that we have the capacity to accept and adjust to these changes, rather than being worn-out or worn-down by them. Our capacity to deal with change is cultivated through building our resilience. As we build our resilience, we develop a reservoir of inner strength that enables us to cope with what comes our way and to favorably adjust to the challenges we face.

A key factor in building resilience is how we think about adversity. The longer we live, the more adversity we inevitably face, so it is critical that we have an approach that empowers us. If we believe we have the psychological strength to cope with stressful events, and if we expect to adapt well in the face of adversity, we move through life with a strong mindset. The reality is that it is not so much the events in our life, as it is our perceived lack of ability to handle those events that makes us anxious.

If we don't have a strong mindset, we can develop it by choosing to frame the way we approach our experiences. We can choose to approach the events we encounter consciously with the intention of growth and as an opportunity to become more self-aware. We can choose to see adversity as a powerful teacher in which we can learn valuable life lessons. Embracing this attitude empowers us to face and accept what comes our way with courage and equanimity.

Accepting our difficulties with courage and being fiercely determined to create something meaningful from them enables us see the possibility in every situation. It helps us to find some silver lining in even the worst of circumstances and to garner wisdom which ultimately could lead to a deeper fulfillment of life. Being determined to find meaning in the conditions that we face allows us to see that what we thought of as a breakdown could actually be the portal to a breakthrough.

Finding the breakthrough in difficult situations requires giving up ways of thinking that haven't worked for us such as worrying, complaining, and taking things personally. Rather than worrying and complaining about the uncontrollable aspects of situations which can leave us feeling helpless, discovering the leap forward requires focusing our time and energy on those facets with which we have some control. Clearly the facet over which we have the most control is our own mind. Choosing to question our stressful thoughts can prevent them from evolving into a full-blown stressful story which can only produce a nightmare.

Believing our stressful stories can lead us to feeling like a victim and trapped in self-pity, which prevents us from seeing beyond our problems and holds us captive to our own misery. Caught in our misery, we tend to keep the self-defeating cycle going by focusing even more excessively on our difficulties causing them to become exaggerated. This detrimental way of thinking perpetuates our suffering and results in a repetition of the same patterns. However, when we question our stressful thoughts, we find that things begin to shift, and we are no longer a prisoner of our own thoughts and habitual behavior.

Engaging in negative, stressful thinking impairs our resilience and leads us to believe that difficult situations are beyond our capability to handle. It also makes us vulnerable to feelings of being overwhelmed. We are then more inclined to focus on negative outcomes and to think pessimistically. We are more likely to deny, blame, and minimize which prevents us from taking accountability. We are also more likely to turn to unhealthy coping mechanisms such as addictions rather than face our difficulties head on.

Aging has the potential to expand our resiliency powers and to help us break free of unhealthy patterns. The confidence and competence we have garnered in solving problems over the years can provide a reservoir of trust enabling us to have faith that we have the ability to surmount rather than succumb. The wisdom of our life experiences offers us the opportunity to see that habits of dwelling on our problems, becoming overwhelmed, or feeling victimized impede our ability to deal with our challenges and to move forward. With the insight and assurance that only experience can bring, we are equipped to handle our difficulties in an empowered way.

Our life experiences have also given us the chance to learn to reconcile ourselves with difficulties that cannot be altered. As we age, we become wise enough to understand that trying to explain the unexplainable is fruitless. We know the question is "What are we going to do about it?" Recognizing that both the actions we take as well as our attitude will affect the outcome of an event, we choose to take steps forward with a positive perspective. We choose to believe that we have the ability to act in ways that help us cope with the unexpected, as well as to engage in choices that lead to our desired goals. With this empowered view, we are liberated from any sense of helplessness and move toward establishing a sense of stability and equilibrium.

In addition to taking action with a positive mindset, maintaining our stability and equilibrium requires the skill of regulating our emotions. Emotional regulation is utilizing our capacity to influence our feelings, instead of being controlled by our emotions like a puppet on a string. Regulating our emotions involves expressing our emotions in a constructive rather than impulsive or hurtful way so that our behavior does not end up at the mercy of our emotions.

Building our resilience requires learning how to become more proficient in navigating emotionally powerful events in our lives rather than feeling totally defenseless in the face of them. Noticing our emotions without making them larger than they need to be, or pushing them away, allows us to find our way through intense situations. As we learn to acknowledge, accept, and learn from the valuable insights our emotions provide, we trust they are bringing to our attention what we need to know. We trust they are offering important information which would only make us stronger and more resilient.

Our most painful emotions show us what we are most resistant to experiencing or changing. When it comes down to it, all the negativity we feel is due to resisting something that is going on in our life. This resistance causes suffering. The more we resist, the more suffering we will experience. If we surrender moment by moment to whatever is happening rather than resisting and fighting against, we find freedom. We also find creative solutions. By surrendering to what is, we open up a space for new opportunities.

Surrender is all too frequently confused with giving up. Giving up can be thought of as slamming the door shut, whereas with surrender we allow doors to open. With surrender we let go of trying to control, deny, or fight the reality of our life. We let go of all those ways of reacting that make life a struggle. With surrender we realize that not only is trying to control everything impossible, it is exhausting.

The process of surrender often leads to a discovery of those parts of our personality that are creating our emotional suffering due to our resistance to what is. The more we surrender, the more those parts of our personality lose power over us, and the more we move into a calm sense of acceptance that offers us peace of mind. We find great freedom when we loosen our grip, surrender, and become more flexible. In fact, one of the most potent ways to counter our resistance to what is showing up in our life is to become flexible.

The essence of resilience is our ability to adapt flexibly—to accept what comes our way with flexibility rather than rigidity, and to meet and recover from setbacks. With flexibility we are able to change course and soldier on. If one door has closed, we walk through the door that is now swinging wide open for us. Thus, we not only bounce back from setbacks rather than being defeated, but we also bounce back stronger and wiser. In fact, if we are resilient, we expect to bounce back and feel confident that we will.

Expecting to bounce back and feeling confident that we will is an optimistic attitude. An optimistic attitude contributes to resiliency. Optimism is the tendency to expect the best possible outcome, and it fills us with an expansive sense of our own power to help shape events. We benefit not only from being optimistic ourselves, but also by surrounding ourselves with optimistic people as resilience develops best in the context of a supportive environment.

Mentally strong people tend to have the support of family and friends who help bolster them up in times of trouble, and who help them feel loved. In fact, the greatest boost to emotional resiliency is to feel loved. There is no substitute for our mental well-being than feeling loved and cared for.

Feeling loved is the one thing we all want. We also have an equally parallel need: the need to love and care for others. Our happiness levels are greatly enhanced when we love and care for others as we have an innate desire to connect. The number of meaningful connections we have with others greatly impacts our emotional well-being and quality of life, as well as our ability to be resilient.

Feeling deeply connected to other people and feeling appreciated by them helps us to feel valued and secure. We can have scores of acquaintances, but if none of our connections feels intimate and meaningful, we will ultimately feel alone. Feelings of loneliness impede our resiliency. Unfortunately, as we age we are increasingly called upon to deal with issues of loneliness as one of the stressors of getting older is multiple losses—loss of spouse, loss of close friends, loss of siblings, and many others.

Loss, in all of its many forms, can be one of the most intense experiences we go through. When we feel loss, we are often not just experiencing the sadness of the current loss, but we are also vulnerable to old emotions that are of similar content being triggered. Our way through the loss, however, is to feel the emotions and then focus on positive steps we can take to elevate our mood. Cutting off from our emotions to avoid pain will only cause further problems and push us away from life itself as we can't selectively numb pain without numbing joy.

We can also become aware of the stressful thoughts behind the feelings and question those thoughts. As we do so, we often find a shift in our perception which results in a change of our feelings, as well as a level of acceptance. Acceptance entails making peace with the loss, letting go, and slowly moving forward with our life.

In many ways, with its cascading losses, aging calls for us to be champions at letting go and continually adapting ourselves to a "new normal." As we adjust to life's endings and beginnings, and accept that all things are in an eternal state of change, we build our resiliency. We accept that loss is written into the fabric of our existence and that we will indeed be faced with its arrival and all the fear it presents.

Resilience involves facing not only our fear of loss, but all of our fears. Overcoming the fears that prevent us from experiencing the joy of life is exceedingly important because we then eliminate the power those fears have over us. Before we can move beyond our fears, we have to recognize and accept them. If we ignore or deny them, we stay stuck and push them into the shadow where they cause an even greater disturbance. Each time we successfully deal with a fear, our resiliency is strengthened.

Mindfulness is a very simple form of meditation that can help us deal with our fears. It essentially involves emotional regulation through attention regulation. Mindful attention to our emotions involves not judging, but observing our emotions when they arise. This can lower our brain's emotional response to anxiety and distress and effectively calm down our amygdala. Even a few weeks of mindfulness practice has been shown to create positive changes in the brain.

Mindfulness is one of the many positive lifestyle choices in which we can engage that help make us more resilient. Any choice we make which adds greater meaning, joy, and depth to our daily life enhances our emotional hardiness. However, the way we think about situations is the greatest boost to our resiliency. Believing that we have the ability to influence the outcome of events, and seeing the events as challenges to master rather than threats to our well-being, gives us a greater sense of confidence and competence. In addition, choosing to consistently sow our minds with new ideas so that we have fresh perspectives leads us to growing inwardly stronger.

Keeping our eyes open for the blessings as well as the beautiful moments along the way enables us to accept the inevitable changes life brings. As we learn to appreciate the ever-changing horizons and the new views each horizon offers, we gain a refreshing outlook and a more resilient spirit. We see that though changes bring challenges, they also contain the potential for growth, as well as the possibility of living happier than we were before they arrived.

6

ACCEPTING OURSELVES UNCONDITIONALLY AND WITH COMPASSION

Self-acceptance and self-compassion are critical to successful aging as they allow us to cope more effectively with the stresses and changes that come our way. There is no substitute for finding the peace and joy that comes from accepting ourselves unconditionally and with compassion.

The need to feel accepted, loved, and understood is at the core of human experience. We can offer these gifts to ourselves. We can open our heart to ourselves. We can choose to infuse our thoughts and actions towards ourselves with love rather than fear. We can choose each moment to treat ourselves as if we were our own best friend.

Self-acceptance and self-compassion are skills that we can nurture. We can learn to hold ourselves with the kindness of a mother holding her child. We can learn how to return to our sense of worth when we get lost in our stories of self-judgment. We can learn how to offer ourselves care when we are suffering. When we practice these skills, feelings of warmth, understanding and gentleness toward ourselves emerge.

31

A powerful way to practice self-acceptance and self-compassion is by becoming our own loving parent. We were all once children, and, no matter what our age, we still have that child dwelling within us. We are constantly being influenced by this inner child whether we are conscious of it or not. Our inner child's fears and insecurities, as well as the joys and feelings of wonder, often unfold into the emotional patterns of our adult lives. As we learn to take our inner child seriously and to consciously communicate with that child, we learn to take care of our needs. Being a supportive, nurturing and encouraging parent to ourselves gives us the strength to deal with the changes life brings and helps to alleviate our suffering.

Most of us are not skilled in listening to the voice of our inner child. And even if we do hear that voice, we have not listened to it without some form of judgment, moralizing, or shaming – all of which discounts our feelings. Learning to become a loving and understanding parent towards our inner child through both our deep listening and internal dialogue can be a gateway to self-acceptance.

The habit of self-acceptance is one of the most important habits we can practice to live a happy life. Self-acceptance is the ability to accept ourselves as we are with all of our strengths and weaknesses instead of focusing on how we wish to be. Such acceptance allows us to let go of our attachment to ideas of perfection and minimizes our tendency to judge and criticize ourselves. It is essentially our way of showing that we approve of ourselves.

Accepting ourselves as we are does not mean we will lose our motivation to change and that we do nothing to improve. Self-acceptance is not opposite to self-improvement, but a fundamental part of it. With self-acceptance we take into account our limitations as we make every effort to further develop ourselves. We embrace whatever we think, feel, or do, even if we don't always like it, and then change and grow into the more ideal person we desire to be.

The practice of fully embracing ourselves as we age runs at a crosscurrent to our culture's prejudice and rejection of older people. This contemptuousness can make finding a sense of acceptance of ourselves difficult when faced with so many negative messages and caricatures of aging. Feelings that are deeply rooted in our society make themselves felt in our inner psychological world. Internalizing these prejudiced attitudes can lead to our own thoughts becoming unkind and wounding. Thus society's attitudes, plus our own private angst about getting old, can undermine our self-acceptance.

However, we can maintain our positive sense of self in the face of the stressors associated with ageist attitudes by not passively accepting these negative stereotypes. We do not have to live our life trapped in these ageist patterns. We can train our mind to think differently about ourselves and the process of aging. We can choose to believe that our self-acceptance can actually increase with age as we become more of our authentic self.

As we choose to become more of our authentic self and thus more self-accepting, we rely less on things outside of ourselves to define us. Our interest in anyone's approval or being perceived as anyone special diminishes. We no longer seek external validation but rather value ourselves and what our experience has taught us. We increasingly kick ageism out of our own head by refusing to assess the worth of ourselves, or anyone else, based on age.

As we confront long-standing patterns of thought and action and move toward greater self-acceptance, it is essential that we have compassion for ourselves. We need to have compassion for how the stereotypes and prejudices of aging have wounded our souls and fueled self-rejection. We need to have compassion for how our competitive, youth-oriented society has fostered feelings of unworthiness leading to negative self-judgment. Extending compassion to ourselves is not only an act of deep kindness to ourselves, but an active expression of acceptance of ourselves just as we are.

The first step in offering compassion is to acknowledge our suffering—to turn towards our emotional discomfort. In fact, self-compassion is a loving response to our suffering. Our society tends to reward being stoic and toughing things out more than it does being kind and nurturing to ourselves. But we need to be able to comfort and care for ourselves the way we naturally desire others to care for us. Self-nurturance needs to be part of our own behavioral repertoire; otherwise, we tend to self-indulge as a way to manage our emotions. Self-indulgent behaviors typically offer pleasure up front but a price to pay later, whereas self-nurturance behaviors create more happiness both immediately and in the long run.

In contrast to self-indulgence, which can be excessive and unhealthy, self-nurturance is the loving care we offer ourselves. It is both pleasurable activities and supportive self-talk. Supportive self-talk is choosing to talk to ourselves in an affirming way. As we do so, we re-write deeply entrenched programming. We learn to praise ourselves rather than criticize ourselves. We become very good at being our own inner ally and having our own back.

Self-nurturance can help us deal with the impact that ageism has played on our self-worth by countering the negative self-talk we have internalized. Even though society gives the message that getting old is grim, the truth is there is only one person who can make us feel good or bad about ourselves—that power lies within us. Regardless of how thick the cultural conditioning is, we get to decide how to respond. However, there is no doubt that resisting the prevailing ageist attitudes requires determination and courage, because even though it may be flying under the proverbial radar, negativity toward aging is culturally pervasive.

Countering the ageism we experience in society by treating ourselves with respect, love and compassion helps prevent our self-worth from suffering. These are gifts we offer ourselves that empower us and give us control over our own life. However, many of us are hesitant to let go of our inner critic. We actually believe we need the inner critic to motivate ourselves. We are afraid we will not do what we need to do if we give up criticizing ourselves. We think that self-criticism will somehow keep us in line and will ensure that we achieve our goals.

The fact is we are more effective when we are kind and constructive with ourselves than when we are critical. We are more successful when we replace self-criticism with self-correction. Allowing our mistakes to give us the opportunity to re-examine our intentions, reconsider our commitments, and adjust our actions can put us on a better path. Accepting that we are imperfect humans living in an imperfect world generates self-compassion.

The ability to soothe and comfort our self with a compassionate response when we make mistakes, as well as when we face the many changes that a long life brings, is invaluable. As we practice comforting ourselves in the way that we comfort others, we become more skillful with offering ourselves compassion. In fact, treating ourselves with the same goodwill and benevolence that we treat others is the heart of self-compassion. When we feel compassion for others, we feel kindness and empathy toward them, and a desire to help reduce their suffering. It is the same when we are compassionate towards ourselves—we turn toward and accept our painful experiences in a kind, loving, non-judgmental way. Rather than defensively avoiding or alienating ourselves from our emotions, we embrace ourselves with kindness and care.

Self-compassion is often confused with self-pity. Self-compassion is about becoming aware of and sitting with our pain, not pitying or indulging ourselves. When we over identify with our suffering, we get locked in the story line of what has happened and we lose our perspective. Then we go down the rabbit hole of self-pity. Learning to observe and be mindful of our thoughts and feelings so that we are not over identified with them, and thus swept away with negative reactivity, is of supreme importance.

Self-compassion, unlike self-pity, helps us to refrain from overreacting and getting caught up in our emotional drama. Rather, it helps us to treat ourselves with kindness and concern when we experience stressful events. This ability is a great asset as we move along our aging journey and navigate the challenges of life. Soothing ourselves with self-compassion and self-acceptance as we weather life's transitions can open the doorway to an unconditional love for ourselves and others as we remember our humanness and connect with the humanity of others.

7

Embracing a New Definition of Beauty

We know that what makes us truly beautiful comes from the heart. We know our spirit is the essence of our beauty. We know that true beauty has very little to do with the symmetry of our face but rather with the way we act and think. We know that when our countenance is aglow with both happiness and virtue, we radiate beauty. Yet all too often beauty is something we strive for rather than see in our essence. Rather than being in touch with the beautiful qualities of our true self, we are more likely to see the ways we don't fit into our culture's narrow, punishing ideal of beauty. This is especially true for women who live in a world in which we are far too often judged on our looks.

The beauty molded by society has not included the aging face and body. This exclusion has set us up to internalize the psychological equation linking youth with beauty. Certainly there are those who are not particularly concerned with their outward appearance and are not invested in this cultural equation. Therefore, this chapter may seem irrelevant to the minority who have not experienced anxiety or sadness over their changing looks. But for those of us who feel impacted by society's all too often definition of beauty as youth, examining that cultural message can be liberating.

Many of us find that aging peacefully and gratefully has not been easy when we have been so culturally conditioned to believe that the attractiveness of youth – a totally transient attribute – is the gateway to happiness and success. This conditioning puts us in the turbulent waters of self-doubt as our bodies begin to change beyond the acceptable societal beauty standard. However, as we begin to realize the pervasiveness and the unreality of the staying forever-young syndrome, we can gently begin to surrender such ideas and offer our aging bodies love and compassion.

As we choose not to buy into society's standards of what is beautiful or attention-worthy, and refuse to believe that youth is the commodity that matters the most, we are on the path to freedom. Freeing ourselves of the psychological equation that equates youth and beauty with the keys to happiness can be challenging but a tremendous liberation. The first step in that liberation is as simple as embracing the idea that quite possibly the opposite is true—that the key to beauty is happiness. When we are happy, we feel connected to ourselves and others. We feel confident, grateful, loving, and purposeful—all attributes which radiate a magnetic beauty.

However, far too often, and especially for women, too much of our happiness is attached to our appearance. This is particularly painful when the current definition of beauty is not very generous. The narrowness of the ever-growing list of unrealistic beauty standards is a detriment to all—not just to older people. Images of perfectly sculpted bodies, flawless skin, wrinkle-free faces, inflated lips and other stereotypical ideals impact us. These societal messages feed the fears of even the young, and make the anticipatory anxiety which aging can generate feel overwhelming. Before we are even old, we may already be fearing what our later years may bring.

Allowing ourselves to make room for a broader, more flexible definition of beauty than the limited perception our culture offers would greatly expand our consciousness and support us in embracing our ever-changing appearance. Expanding our idea of beauty to make it more inclusive and to embrace all the infinite forms of beauty—different ages, colors, sizes, shapes, and heritages—disrupts the prevailing attitudes and challenges the status quo. And doing so empowers each and every one of us. Through embracing our own meaningful images of beauty and refusing to believe we are inadequate unless we present ourselves in certain culturally sanctioned ways, we create a break-through for all.

With images of idealized beauty bombarding us daily, it is easy to forget that beauty is arbitrary and its ideals are ever changing. It can also vary significantly from one culture to another. In fact, no culture or concept could ever truly define beauty as the experience of beauty is so vast and unique that it defies a simplistic or narrow description. Yet we take our images of how we should look to be the truth, and they become a compelling reality which takes most of our attention. We are too easily convinced that without the culturally defined youthful beauty we do not measure up. This can impact our self-esteem, particularly for women whose physical beauty historically has been the major source of their personal power.

Sadly, the number one domain in which the majority of women invest their self-esteem and obtain a sense of personal power is through their appearance. This way of thinking comes primarily from harboring the illusion that with beauty we have the power to get the love we need. Thus we keep searching for ways to be more beautiful because we think that would make us more lovable. Attaching our lovability to our appearance, we unknowingly use our appearance as an exchange for love.

If we no longer feel we can use our appearance as collateral, our sense of safety which comes from feeling loved is jeopardized. This makes the physical changes that aging brings especially painful as the major area in which we have learned to get our self-worth appears to get challenged. Though it requires a firm resolve, we can choose to move beyond the false belief that our worth is determined by our physical appearance.

We also get to decide how we will talk to ourselves when we look in the mirror and see a face no longer young. Whether our inner voice will be self-critical and shaming or loving and accepting is our choice. Unfortunately, when we look in the mirror, all too often we have in our minds the perfect image—a perfect image which causes us to be critical and shaming. Our minds get busy judging and finding fault with our appearance and assuming that others do the same. We tend to believe that everyone agrees with our negative opinion of ourselves. We then try to look more and more perfect because we believe the only way to eliminate that critical inner voice is to be perfect enough.

The good news is that each time we are able to be less judgmental toward ourselves or others, we become more liberated. Each time we summon the courage to challenge the social biases and refuse to allow false images of how we should look to run our life, we find freedom. These positive choices improve our self-esteem. And with every choice we take to improve our self-esteem, we improve our body image. The truth is that body image is more closely tied to self-esteem than to external signs of beauty. When self-esteem is high, body image is generally positive.

One of the most powerful ways to improve our self-esteem is to be our authentic self. Being our authentic self is living our life in alignment with our own deepest beliefs and values.

Living authentically makes us an example of a beautiful person, for to be in the presence of someone who is authentically and unapologetically themselves, and comfortable with their perfect imperfections, is to be in the presence of beauty.

When we have a rock-solid identity as to who we truly are, beautifying and adorning ourselves can be fun. We can playfully spruce ourselves up with objects when we are totally clear that we are not an object. The problem with any way we beautify ourselves exists only when we feel inferior or inadequate without doing so. We have every right to pursue and enhance our outward beauty. The issue isn't so much the personal choices we make to enhance our appearance, but the consciousness in which we do it.

The practice of enhancing our appearance and desiring a youthful one is certainly not new as the search for the fountain of youth and beauty has been taking place for centuries. Although we resemble our ancestors and other cultures in our concern about appearance, there is a difference in the degree of concern. Advances in technology, and in particular the rise of social media, has caused normal concerns about how we look to become obsessions. In today's media-saturated world in which we are bombarded with images of what we should look like—and what we fail to look like—the over-valuation of physical attractiveness is more intense than ever.

Putting a halt to breeding a society that equates external appearance with intrinsic value is up to us. A vital starting point is to teach our children to reject the notion of an exclusive beauty standard, as well as to provide them with resourceful ways to deal with a world encased in artificial standards of beauty. As we teach and model for them that our value comes from our character and attributes—not our appearance—we are the living, breathing proof that beauty is not limited in any way, shape, or form. Additionally, we need to acknowledge our own prejudice around aging and appearance, our own internalized biases such as "being too old" or seeing others as "too old," which adds to the dilemma.

Thankfully, not everyone has accepted or internalized the socially sanctioned standards of beauty. There are strong-minded individuals who have been brave enough to challenge the norm and live their own brand of beauty. They show us that the definition of beauty is broader than we have been trained to think. Whether they are plus-sized or albino models, people campaigning against the beauty industry, founders of body image movements, or just everyday individuals boldly living their own truth, they are confronting the myth that our value depends on the attractiveness of our bodies.

The maturing of society has the potential to alter the unrealistic standards that have plagued us for so long. With the population of those over sixty expected to double in the next thirty years, eyes will get accustomed to seeing images of mature beauty. New visions of what makes a person beautiful will persist as the older generation continues to grow in numbers. As our vision of beauty changes, this will help us develop a more accepting relationship with our appearance and body, and the by-product will be a more loving and appreciative relationship with ourselves.

When we appreciate ourselves we are able to see that what is truly beautiful about us is our resilience, kindness, generosity, and infinite capacity to love, often in the face of great struggles. We are able to see that every time we open our heart and surrender to love we are expressing the beauty of our spirit and adding positive energy to the world. As the beauty of our spirit continues to unfold, the more beauty we will express, and the more profound beauty we will see in the simplest of things.

If we practice seeing the spirit of each other—seeing each other as souls instead of bodies—our ideals of beauty change even more dramatically. We then understand that our appearance simply clothes the essence of who we are. Shedding the cloak of misidentification of ourselves as only our physical body liberates us, and we begin to see everything through new eyes. We will feel as if the filters have been removed and we are no longer wearing glasses with distorted lenses. We come to know who we truly are.

Knowing Who We Truly Are

As we look into the bathroom mirror examining the signs of age and feeling our insecurities swell, it might be difficult to remember who we truly are. We may forget that though our appearance has changed, nothing essential about us has changed at all. We may forget that we are losing nothing real by getting older. In the grip of seeing our physical changes, our anxiety can block us from connecting with our true essence which is untouched by time.

Becoming so identified with our physical form and losing touch with our formless essence is easy to do. We have been conditioned to see ourselves through our physical packaging—through ego-centered eyes. The eyes of the ego see an identity defined by our physical body and all the different beliefs we have acquired. This mind-made sense of who we are—this mental construct—becomes our self-image.

Most of us have spent a life time building up our ego's self-image and spending our energy defending, protecting and maintaining this image. We have grown up trying to shape our self-image around whatever culture deemed to be most valuable because we all wanted to be desired, loved, and valued. We then became trapped within this erroneous identification of the person we created and believed this image to be who we are. We identified ourselves with the mask rather than our true self behind it. One of the gifts of aging is that it can act as a displacing of this mask and as an opening to our true self.

As our bodies begin to feel and reflect the physical changes that come with our advancing years, aging can be an assault to our ego. This blow to our ego offers us the opportunity to know who we truly are and spark our awakening. As we awaken, we come to know that the real us is not our body, our mind, or our personality. The real us is that which is aware of every thought, feeling, sensation, and insight that we experience. The real us is the presence which is watching—the witnessing awareness which is pure consciousness.

There are many words used to point to this pure consciousness, the essence of who we are—soul, awareness, presence, eternal being, infinite self are but a few of the names. But whatever term we use, nothing matters more in life than an awareness and connection to this presence. This presence is the being part of ourselves as human beings. This presence is the timeless, changeless witness—our spark of the one universal intelligence which flows through all of life.

Without an awareness of this presence, we become identified with our outer shell and the dimension of form which keeps us trapped in our ego. This leads to suffering. In fact, the more unaware we are of this animating presence within, the more we suffer. Our true liberation is knowing and living connected to this presence. Living connected to this presence, we become increasingly aware that we are more than a temporary form in the universe. As a result, much of the confusion and unhappiness in our life falls away. By shedding our identification with our physical form and ego selves, we wake up to the source of our true power and to the pure love that we essentially are. This pure love and power is like the sunshine that is always present behind the clouds.

Yet as the term so aptly expresses, we are human beings —human is the material aspect of us, and being is the non-material. Being human, we must deal with all the things that living in this world brings, as well as those aspects of our personality that are rooted in fear. Utilizing our conscious capacity to align with the being part of us as we navigate daily life and the journey of our advancing years gives us the strength to face our fears, and to function with greater clarity and purpose. But until we align with this deeper aspect of our self, our personality will be driven by the fears of our ego.

Aligning with this transcendent dimension of ourselves is the opening to true happiness. Our desires then come from our deeper self rather than our ego, and we no longer mistake what we have, what we do, or what we look like for our identity. Rather than looking to the achievement of our goals or other externals to bring us happiness, or to enhance our sense of self, we find joy and meaning in each step of our journey.

As we continue our passage from mid-life to old age, we may find ourselves leaving our acquisitive goals behind and learning to simply be more present for the moment. During this stage, while our outer life may be subsiding, our inner life can be flourishing. In addition, we may find a great liberation in disentangling our sense of self from all the things with which we had become identified. This disentanglement involves learning to witness our body, mind, and emotions without identifying with them. We become the observer—the witness—and not the observed.

Being the observer rather than the observed is an opportunity to expand beyond our human conditioning. If we open to and surrender to its powerful potential, being the observer of what is happening in the world of form is an opportunity to unfold to our true nature as well as to meet aging in an empowering way. We begin to see the process of aging through the eyes of the eternal being that we truly are rather than through the eyes of our ego. We understand that who we really are, beyond the illusory ego self, is changeless. We begin to know ourselves as souls rather than skin encapsulated egos.

To embrace aging as a path of awakening to who we truly are is perhaps the most important meaning we can give to this phase of our life. In fact, the journey of life is ideally about awakening to the eternal being that we are. Knowing who we are, knowing that which is real and eternal but not seen or touched, is intuitively discerned. Being still, being silent, being receptive and holding a listening attitude is the way. In stillness and solitude we meet that part of us that is eternal.

Our later years can offer us the gifts of stillness and solitude and can be the most spiritually meaningful time of our life. As our body ages and loses some of its youthful strength, our soul can get richer and stronger. However, too often when we look at older people, all we see is the disturbing image of a frail and worn body. We have to teach ourselves to see beyond the mask of aging. Our lives will change dramatically when we begin to see each other through soul-centered eyes and allow our fundamental relationship to be soul to soul. As we do so, we increasingly find ourselves without any sense of separation between ourselves and the rest of the world—we feel our oneness with all others. This experience of oneness makes us even more aware of the times when we fall back into our conditioned sense of self which is a limited, isolated sense of existence.

As we allow our spiritual growth to become our focus and purpose in life, we begin to drop our limitations and fearful beliefs which we've been carrying around for so long like a heavy sack of rocks on our back. The reservoir of accumulated negative feelings which have made us miserable, and is the basis of many of our illnesses, begins to fall away. We find our negative emotions being replaced with love and acceptance and our erroneous beliefs supplanted with spiritual knowledge and wisdom, which greatly accelerate our spiritual growth.

We can use the process of aging, as well as all of life's experiences, to further our spiritual evolution which means to wake up to who we truly are. Waking up to our true self transforms our consciousness—the state of our awareness. Transforming our consciousness is the most important thing we can do for ourselves and for the world as our consciousness determines the overall way that we perceive the world and our place in it. Our consciousness determines the way we treat ourselves and others.

Transforming our consciousness begins by paying attention to the thoughts, feelings, and behaviors that are present in our everyday lives. It begins by paying attention to the present moment and being fully present to our habits. As we break free from our negative habits through our choice to connect with the greater intelligence within us, we deconstruct the old and create anew. We allow our essential goodness, our innate wisdom, and our compassion to unfold and to navigate our lives. We allow ourselves to be the divine creators that we truly are and, ultimately, unleash our true greatness.

9

CREATING YOUR UNIQUE PERSONAL VISION AND PURPOSE

The possibility is vast for our later years to be infused with a larger purpose, passion, and growth than we have ever known. However, the myths about being older may silently influence our belief in this possibility as well as our choices in this particularly fertile period of our life. For example, an underlying message seems to exist in our mainstream culture that after we have arrived at a certain age, we have already reached the pinnacle of our success. Yet, in many ways, all the life experiences we have accumulated can be a launching pad into the most fulfilling phase of our life in which we express our creativity to an even greater degree and significantly contribute to the lives of others.

Challenging constricting and limiting myths is essential as our expectations influence the outcomes we experience. The odds that our later years will be a great opportunity for growth and creative expression is appreciably enhanced if we expect them to be. In fact, our later years can be the most creative period in our life as creativity can grow rather than diminish

51

with maturity. This is in part due to the fact that as we get older we tend to have less of a need for acceptance, a greater tendency to ignore social expectations, and an increased ambition to speak our mind—all traits of highly creative people.

As we embrace the truth that growing older is rich with potential, we often discover that dormant desires are reignited within us. We may also notice new aspirations yearning to be born, with the parts of ourselves that have been the least developed calling to us the loudest. Whether those aspirations involve cultivating a beautiful garden, composing masterpieces, designing works of art, inventing unique gadgets, traveling to exotic places, finishing marathons or a host of other stimulating endeavors, the opportunity to express our creativity and launch our dreams is ours to pursue.

Inspired people throughout history have flourished and enjoyed their greatest fulfillment in their later years. We can do the same. Choosing to believe that age doesn't prohibit us from experiencing the gratification of living our dreams and knowing the joy of a purpose-filled life calls for boldness. And boldness requires ignoring age labels. Transcending stereotypical labels, by doing the things we want to do when and where we want to do them, is enormously liberating. As we refuse to define ourselves by the category of age, we no longer decide that we are too old to do something before we truly are.

Mental attitudes of feeling old which may have been lurking in our mind drop away when we are infused with enthusiasm and positive expectancy as we explore new paths. We realize that staying young psychologically means not surrendering the passion, excitement, and creativity we enjoyed in our younger years. We understand that our inner life and curiosity are the keys to our emotional youthfulness. Staying wide-eyed about the world and maintaining our child-like curiosity is critical to thriving at every stage of life. With a curious mind, there are always new things to attract our attention which prevent our lives from becoming dull or boring.

Curiosity has been the driving force behind most discoveries, adventures, and inventions in the history of humankind. It is a form of intrinsic motivation, propelling us to learn and explore new things as well as generating enthusiasm. This enthusiasm allows us to experience our life as an adventurous quest to discover, learn, and grow which makes us more willing to leave the familiar and take risks, even if those risks move us out of our comfort zone. Though coming out of our comfort zone requires risking more, it is where aliveness and vitality abide, and where new rewards await us.

Establishing meaningful intentions supports us in coming out of our comfort zone. Our intentions are our commitment to take action, and they create a sense of positive anticipation. They are powerful navigators directing our attention and energy. They are also the fuel to reach our goals and dreams as they keep us focused. Intentions help us align our habitual mind with the purposes we want to fulfill, thus empowering us to take the necessary steps to make our dreams a reality.

When we focus on meaningful intentions which are in alignment with our sense of purpose, we feel better—and, thus life, gets better. Negative emotions become less frequent and more fleeting when they do occur as our intentions uplift our emotions and energize us to take action. As we take positive action, we become renewed and regenerated. We find our curiosity about life to be expanding and our imagination flourishing.

The power of our imagination is the ultimate mind power. It plays a major role in how we experience all aspects of life. We cannot escape from the creative power of our imagination as we are continually using it every minute of our life. The question to be asked is whether we are using it to create the life for which we yearn. Using our imagination as a powerful creative tool to shape the life we desire necessitates that we focus on the reality we want to experience through the use of our thoughts, words, and actions. Doing so gives us a sense of anticipation and aliveness as to what our future holds. Utilizing the power of our imagination also gives us the ability to look at any situation from a different point of view, thus allowing us to shift our limiting beliefs about what is possible. As we come to expand our sense of possibilities, we begin to move forward in exciting ways.

Regardless of our age, we need to feel as though we are advancing in the direction of worthwhile endeavors. One of the characteristics of young people is that they are typically looking forward which is why they are often viewed as more advantaged psychologically. Having pleasurable things to anticipate keeps us enthusiastic about life. When we do not feel we have anything gratifying to anticipate, we begin to decline both mentally and physically. We begin to feel old and pessimistic. Through a pessimistic lens, all we see ahead is less time, diminished status, declining health, fewer opportunities, and waning attractiveness. We become sad adults aching at the loss of youth and fearfully turning away from our future by seeing it only as a downward spiral.

Establishing purposes and intentions that fulfill us and offer us a strong reason for waking up in the morning prevents any sense of a downward spiral. To the contrary, we find ourselves imbued with the passion that having a purpose brings. Living a life of purpose doesn't necessarily mean to inhabit a busy world of doing and achieving, but to be involved with experiences that feel meaningful and pleasurable. As we do so, we recapture that feeling of wonder and forward-looking excitement that we had in our younger years.

While looking forward to the next adventure that life holds brings much optimism and joy to our life, savoring where we are and what we have is essential for our happiness. Our sense of aliveness is expanded as we live in the actual present while imaging our possible future with a sense of gratitude and fullness. When we are wholly present for the deep satisfaction that living in the moment brings, we experience the greatest joy life has to offer. This often happens when we are completely absorbed in something that matters to us such as working on a project, playing a sport, reading a book, being with someone we love, or any other activity in which we are totally present.

When we were younger, things that mattered to us were often determined by their ability to help us achieve, to generate money, to be well-known, or to attract others. As we get older, our priorities often change as visions that once were dazzling from a distance don't look as glamourous up close. We may find that at this stage of our life we want inner peace more than we want to win the trophies. We may find ourselves past the point of striving for additional accolades or possessions, and searching for something more deeply fulfilling.

As we direct our attention toward those things that truly matter to us rather than being distracted by the superficial, we are better able to focus on that which we want to bring forth in the world. We let go of old dreams so that we can create new ones. We choose to become involved with life in more gratifying ways. As we summon the courage to examine and possibly relinquish how we have been defining ourselves and living our life, we make new commitments. This process may require changes or sacrifices that seem uncomfortable or unpleasant, but which more than often lead to something greater and more fulfilling.

Letting go of old identities and our familiar world can be very difficult and frightening, particularly when new ones aren't yet clearly defined. However, we can allow our fear to be a force for creativity and growth, and for bringing us closer to living a truly authentic life. As we choose to live a life that is more authentic, we are naturally happier and thus impact the world around us in a more positive way. Impacting the world in a positive way—making a difference to someone or something—gives us that sense of fulfillment for which we long and brings us immense joy.

Most of us yearn to make our lives about something more than our own comforts and successes. We know that our fulfillment is greatly expanded when we dedicate our actions not only to benefit ourselves and those we love, but also to all beings. In fact, we are the happiest when we are of service to something larger than ourselves. One of the greatest opportunities of a longer life is that we have more time to give back – to make the world a better place through our inspired action. As we discover the place where the world's needs intersect with our passion, the potential for our contribution to the world is magnified.

Creating a life that will allow us to contribute to the well-being of our world in ways that are in line with our talents and affinities fills us with a sense of purpose. We all want to feel purposeful, to feel our life has meaning, and to fulfill our desires. When we do so, we feel better. When we feel better, we treat other people better, and this produces a ripple effect that spreads out to everyone around us. Each of us has a circle of people whose lives we can help improve. When we work to improve the lives of others, we indirectly elevate our own life in the process.

If we can perceive each moment and every passing year of our life as an opportunity to give and grow, aging can be experienced as a wondrous gift. It is a gift that gives us time to open our hearts even wider so that we become even more willing to help and more accommodating. As we do so, our hearts are expanded, our consciousness is elevated, and we evolve. This personal evolution can be described as our spiritual journey. In fact, aging has the potential to be the most pronounced stage of our spiritual journey.

Our spiritual journey involves examining our inner world. As we look inward, we can discover our unresolved issues that keep us unaware or blocked from living our potential and most importantly, from knowing our essential loving nature. We then have the opportunity to resolve those issues. This may mean revisiting our past in a compassionate and healing way and rewriting any demoralizing stories we may have about the past that are a barrier to our ability to live and love as freely as we desire. We can see that as architects of our own life, the past has given us material with which to work. We have a choice to make use of everything that we have experienced, to see our past as one big bank account giving us our present richness and wisdom.

Regardless of the direction we take from this day forward, nothing we have experienced is wasted. Everything was simply grist for the mill preparing us to awaken to our true authentic self. The more awake we become, the more all of our past is accepted and appreciated. We understand that we can offer the wisdom we have garnered from our life experiences as a service to the world. A profound state of gratitude for all that we have encountered, and for the gift of our life, can be our overriding emotion until we are ready to depart this earthly journey.

10

Making Peace with our Mortality

As our passing birthdays and changing bodies steadily declare the realities of our aging, a heightened awareness of the time we have left on this earthly journey grows. We find ourselves waking up more intensely to our mortality. Taking stock of our life and being at peace with the inevitable death of our physical body is a crucial part of our life's journey. The increased sense of our mortality which grows with each passing birthday doesn't have to take the pleasure out of the coming years, however. Rather than allowing the realization of our limited time to be an underlying source of anxiety, it can be a catalyst for cutting through the inauthentic, superficial, and meaningless aspects of our life to reveal what really matters.

Reflecting upon the inevitability of our death can be a strong motivator to sort out our priorities and to get our affairs in order which is a loving and wise thing to do both for ourselves and others. Getting our affairs in order can give us a sense of relief even if we have many years of a healthy life ahead of us. Taking the time to organize things related to our personal life is also a great act of lovingkindness toward those we will leave behind. If we do not place our affairs in order, our loved ones will pay a heavy price both financially and emotionally.

Facing our mortality may also compel us to confront and resolve any unfinished issues from our past. Engaging in the inner work necessary to come to terms with our past and any regrets we may have allows us to leave this life peacefully and to make our transition with an unburdened soul. Facing our mortality presents the opportunity for emotional healing so that we are more caring and forgiving of ourselves and others. It can move us to make peace with our life and to embrace and honor each moment more deeply.

Though there is value in confronting our death, and bringing the topic of death out into the open, we tend to avoid even thinking or talking about it. A conversation about death is often thought of as a morbid and fear-invoking experience even though our physical death is an inevitable and natural part of life. There seems to be a strange superstition that if you talk about death, you invite it closer. Death is shunned as a legitimate subject in polite circles as it tends to conjure up strong feelings, and even talking about death is often considered depressing.

In our culture we try to ignore death by keeping it largely out of sight and out of mind. Our anxiety is revealed by the fact that even corpses are dressed up, embalmed and given a make-over so as to look like they are merely sleeping. One of the reasons given for this ritual is that making a dead body look as if it is sleeping enables the bereaved to process the death psychologically. However, much of our difficulty in processing death has been due to our learned responses.

We have, for the most part, been conditioned to view death as something to fear and even a tragedy. We have turned the process of dying and death into a frightful experience—even an encroachment upon life—rather than seeing it as a sacred and necessary part of life. This unnatural view of death is unhealthy and fails to serve us as individuals or as a society. Our failure to ponder our own fear of death is an important reason why we have found it so difficult to be of greater assistance to the dying and the bereaved. We avoid that which we fear.

Our fear around death seems to be in part natural as well as in part a result of a learned reaction. We innately have a drive to survive. In that respect, the fear of death is natural and valuable as it is part of our "fight or flight" mechanism that has evolved over millions of years. The physical responses produced by the fight or flight mechanism are intended to help us survive by preparing us to either run for our life or fight for our life. In that sense, the fear of death is a helpful evolutionary motivation as it alerts us to take action to survive. However, we are not created to spend our lives in anxious preparation over what may come.

Anxiety—whether about death or other life experiences—is an emotion that looks to the future as it is wrapped up in how things might go. It results in unproductive thought patterns known as catastrophizing which ultimately generates even more negative thought patterns. The majority of the time things do not turn out to be as unpleasant as we imagined them to be. Simply thinking differently, as well as talking about our fears, often loosens the grip that anxiety has on us. It also allows us to adopt a healthier perspective.

Adopting a healthier and less fearful perspective of death empowers us and enables us to function with greater equanimity. There are many perspectives we can take to come to terms with our mortality. One such perspective is a spiritual context in which there is the belief that death is not an end or extinction of life, but is a change in existence in which the soul passes to another realm. Spiritual teachers and mystics throughout history have taught this conviction, referring to our earthly life as but a parenthesis in eternity—that this life experience is only a part of our overall eternal life. The message of these revered teachers is that physical birth and death are but episodic incidents which occur during our journey through space and time.

Another way of stating this idea that death is not the end is to think of our physical body like a garment, a shell covering our eternal soul. Within this spiritual perspective, dying is viewed as merely dropping this shell wherein our external identities are stripped away and only our essence remains. In other words, our personality was born on a certain date and it will die on a certain date, but there is a part of us that existed prior to our birth and will live beyond our death. If we see our life journey against the backdrop of being the eternal souls that these spiritual teachings declare that we are, chances are our anxieties about death are dissipated.

Science also has a language that tells us that our essence has no end as it explains that everything is made up of energy. In fact, we could be described as a field of congealed energy. Energy is the building block of all matter and can neither be created nor destroyed. Energy does not die—it simply transforms. Therefore, it appears that science is beginning to confirm what spiritual masters have been teaching—that we are not just skin encapsulated egos.

The theories of consciousness which come from various religions, philosophy and some corners of science reflect another perspective which supports the eternality of our essence. These theories hold that we are pure consciousness currently focused in a physical dimension and we return to pure consciousness when we die. According to many modern day scientists, as well as the mystics and sages since antiquity, our essence is this pure consciousness—the omniscient, omnipresent, all pervasive substance behind all existence both seen and unseen. Throughout human history sages and philosophers have referred to this universal consciousness as God.

Whether we believe our essence is extinguished with our final breath, or whether we believe there is something more on the other side, embracing a philosophy of life that is meaningful for us helps us view death with trust, calmness and equanimity. The stories we tell ourselves about what happens after death greatly influence our reactions to the thought of death. A worldview that holds us steady when facing our physical impermanence is essential for our well-being. Since we have an absence of evidence either way, perhaps we could speculate that something wonderful happens after death. After all, it makes sense to choose something that comforts us.

Embracing a comforting view of death enables us to move more gracefully through all the endings that life presents. The longer we live the more endings we will experience. These endings are the smaller deaths we encounter throughout our lives. Moving through these smaller deaths with dignity and grace can be a practice to surrendering to our own physical impermanence with equanimity.

No doubt the saddest and hardest part of aging is the loss of those we love. We may find ourselves time and again having to redirect ourselves back to the path of living after a tremendous loss and deep grief. Mourning plays an important role in this process. Mourning our losses frees up a space in which new experiences and qualities can develop. We can move through the grieving process while keeping our loss in perspective— honoring the natural role that death plays in life. We can find comfort in the fact that we all go through the same thresholds of life—birth and death.

Learning to consciously let go is invaluable preparation for dealing with the inevitable losses that accompany both aging and death. Learning to let go allows us to get a different perspective on a situation rather than resisting and struggling. Resisting and struggling contain a great amount of fear. Breaking free of this fear requires looking at the judgments and assumptions which we are making. Questioning the beliefs which generate fear is an important first step in moving beyond them.

By summoning the courage to dive into our fears and our notions about death and dying, we can learn to accept death as a natural part of our human experience. We can wisely move toward those anxieties which trouble us—whether death or any other issue—so that they do not remain underground and interfere with our enjoyment of life. Confronting and making peace with our fears rather than covering them up serves our emotional well-being.

While death is inescapable, our attitudes and beliefs around death are quite negotiable. If we can overcome the fear of death, we may notice other fears falling away. We may find that when we aren't afraid to die, we aren't afraid to really live because we have a sense that nothing can truly harm us, not even death.

Reflecting upon death ends up being not so much about how we die but how we live. When we were young, we had that delicious sense of endless tomorrows with endless possibilities, full of the magic of potential. As we age, our life would take on that same magical quality if we could truly learn to live every day as if it were our last and every moment as a gift. Being rooted in the ability to see ourselves and others with the awareness of our impermanence can wake us up to truly experiencing each moment of our precious time together. It can wake us up to more fully appreciating each opportunity for connection and love.

A common sentiment expressed by many near-death survivors is a heightened appreciation for relationships and loving other people, and a decreased emphasis on material things.

These survivors report returning from such an experience with a new set of values and behaviors that seem to genuinely make them happier and more fulfilled. Even those who reported living with a block toward openness had an awakening experience which catalyzed within them a deep desire for intimacy and connection. It also catalyzed within them a determination to live life on their own terms.

The more we feel we have lived life on our own terms and made our dreams come true, the more prepared we are for that unknown time when death comes calling. Perhaps the greatest sting of death is that of not having used our time the way we would have most desired. Facing the possibility of our death if we feel we have not truly lived can shake us to the core of our being. In fact, what many people fear actually isn't death. They fear they have not lived a fulfilling life. The good news is that even if we haven't yet lived the life we wanted, we can still shift our priorities. Change is always possible. We can change so that at the end we can feel that we have led a full, meaningful and satisfying life.

We can change in any way we feel necessary so that we die with a happy and peaceful mind. Pondering our death allows us to be inspired to live what time we have in such a way as to give ourselves these gifts, and to live our life with meaning and purpose. Facing our mortality can serve as a reminder to use our talents to make our unique contribution to the world and to use our remaining time in ways that fulfill our heart.

Reflecting upon our mortality can stir us to love immeasurably with the awareness that nothing can contribute greater to making our life well-lived. If we want to bequeath a valuable legacy, we must keep in mind that people long remember how loved and valued they feel when in our presence. We must remember the power of love to heal and unite.

In the end, the only things we can say about death for certain is that it is a mystery, it will come, and it is the great equalizer as it is the one thing we all must face. Chances are that when we face the final moments of our life, we will find that our greatest treasures are the tender and heartfelt moments we shared. We will know unquestionably that love is the greatest gift of all—the answer to all that our hearts desire.

Acknowledgment

I am deeply grateful to Mary Beth Gumbart whose superb talent, support, and generosity guided me on every page.

About the Author

Sheryl Towers is an author, speaker, workshop facilitator and life coach. For over two decades she has inspired people to live with purpose, passion, and genuine happiness through her popular keynotes and seminars. She is the founder of Life Enrichment Skills, a company committed to empowering organizations and individuals to achieve peak efficiency and performance, and has served as a consultant to leaders of business, government, and education in the areas of organizational excellence, performance coaching and leadership effectiveness.

Sheryl received her Master of Liberal Studies degree from Mercer University in the area of psychology. She is the author of three books, *Seeds of Success: Nurturing the Greatness within You*, *Transforming Your Life: Moving from Fear to Love, Joy, and Abundance*, and most recently, *Embracing a New Vision of Aging*.

Sheryl is dedicated to helping people live more empowered, fulfilling, and joy-filled lives.

Visit her online at sheryltowers.com.

Also Available From

Sheryl Towers

Seeds of Success
  Nurturing the Greatness Within You

Transforming Your Life
  Moving from Fear to Love, Joy, and Abundance

Also Available From

WordCrafts Press

Pressing Forward
  by April Poynter

Geezer Stories
  by Laura Mansfield

Morning Mist: *Stories from the Water's Edge*
  by Barbie Loflin

Chronicles of a Believer
  by Don McCain

Illuminations
  by Paula K. Parker & Tracy Sugg

A Scarlet Cord of Hope
  by Sheryl Griffin

www.wordcrafts.net

CPSIA information can be obtained
at www.ICGtesting.com
Printed in the USA
BVHW04*1513290718
522886BV00002B/5/P